FROM PMS TO SNAKEBITE...

The herb black cohosh has been used to treat a variety of health problems, but is perhaps most appreciated for the relief it brings to those troubled by complications of menopause—cramps, headaches, hot flashes, emotional upsets—without the problems presented by other approaches, such as hormone replacement.

ABOUT THE AUTHOR

A graduate of Southern Methodist University, where he received the Sigma Delta Chi Outstanding Graduate Award, Frank Murray is Editorial Director of *Let's Live!* magazine. He is author or coauthor of 29 books on health and nutrition, including *Happy Feet* and *The Big Family Guide to All the Minerals*.

Remifemin:
Herbal Relief for Menopausal Symptoms

The safe, natural alternative to hormonal and surgical treatment

Frank Murray

Keats Publishing, Inc.   New Canaan, Connecticut

Remifemin: Herbal Relief for Menopausal Symptoms is intended solely for informational and educational purposes, and not as medical advice. Please consult a medical or health professional if you have questions about your health.

REMIFEMIN: HERBAL RELIEF FOR MENOPAUSAL SYMPTOMS

Copyright © 1996 by Frank Murray

All Rights Reserved

No part of this book may be reproduced in any form without the written consent of the publisher.

ISBN: 0-87983-764-0

Printed in the United States of America

Keats Good Health Guides™ are published by
Keats Publishing, Inc.
27 Pine Street (Box 876)
New Canaan, Connecticut 066840-0876

CONTENTS

Introduction 7
What Is Menopause? 8
Hot Flashes 16
Vaginal Dryness 20
Osteoporosis 22
Heart Disease 25
Insomnia 26
Headaches 26
The Pros and Cons of Estrogen Replacement Therapy 28
Black Cohosh for Menopause 33
Clinical Studies 36
Other Uses for Remifemin 46

INTRODUCTION

Throughout history, menopause, the end of a woman's capacity to bear children, has been associated with decline and death. Partly this is because people used to die younger, and menopause was too often really near the end of life; and the feeling that women were to be valued mainly for the children they produced, and the physical and emotional discomforts that often accompanied the "change of life," contributed to this negative outlook.

As Bernadine Healy, M.D. points out in *A New Prescription for Women's Health,* things have changed. "Our daughters will grow up in a world filled with vigorous, most assuredly alive and active menopausal women. About 35 million women living in America now have gone through or are going through menopause; 90 percent of all women alive today will live through menopause. In fact, most American women can look forward to another 30 years of life after menopause. If menopause is a problem, then every woman has a problem. Seen in this light, the absurdity of this negative attitude becomes clear. As the generation caught between our mothers' perspectives and our daughters' reality, we may have to periodically remind ourselves of this truism."

Although many women pass through menopause with few complications, other women find that their lives are miserable. A healthful diet, exercise, little alcohol, no smoking, etc., often lessen these side effects. For generations, herbalists have recommended a variety of herbs to minimize the health problems that arise during and after menopause. This book concentrates on only one of these: black cohosh or *Cimicifuga racemosa*. It is available in an over-the-counter preparation called Remifemin.

For women with severe problems relating to menopause, it is best to see a holistic practitioner or gynecologist to get professional advice about the various problems.

WHAT IS MENOPAUSE?

Before this century, menopause was a virtual mystery to most physicians, because women seldom lived past the age of 50, a few years before the average onset of menopause, explains Robert M. Giller, M.D., in *Natural Prescriptions*. As women lived longer, doctors—usually males—denied that menopause was anything but a psychological problem, and tranquilizers were often the accepted treatment.

Today most women are familiar with the well-known symptoms of menopause: hot flashes, headaches, sleep disturbances and changes in sexual function and desire. But there are other, long-term results of menopause that are the source of much controversy. At the heart of this controversy is whether menopause and its physical changes should be viewed as a natural event to be endured (or simply ignored by the many women who experience few symptoms), or whether it is an evolutionary mistake that can be corrected by the use of drugs.

"Menopause, which usually occurs around the age of 50 (others say as early as 36 or as late as the sixties, but generally between 44 and 53), is, like puberty, a dramatic change in a woman's body," Giller says. "At menopause, the ovaries, which have been releasing eggs since puberty, shut down and stop producing the hormone estrogen. Of course, if a woman has had her ovaries removed surgically, she will experience menopause immediately, due to the reduction in estrogen, no matter what her age. Menopause does not happen overnight; for most women the process will play out over one to five years with gradually diminishing menstrual periods. During this time the amount of estrogen decreases, and it's this decrease in estrogen that causes the typical symptoms of menopause."

The first sign of menopause for most women is irregular periods. The cycle may shorten or lengthen; the menstrual flow may increase or decrease. A woman can actually be fertile even when she has been without a period for a year. But, after a woman experiences irregular periods for a year to five years, menstruation will stop.

"A year to a year and a half before a woman's period ends, she may experience hot flashes, during which her temperature will rise and fall as much as nine degrees," Giller notes. "These flashes may be accompanied by sweating, heart palpitations, nausea and, not surprisingly, anxiety. Hot flashes can contribute to insomnia; some women complain of waking frequently and having to change damp bedclothes. And some women also notice irritability, headaches, short-term memory loss, lack of sexual desire and inability to concentrate. Some of these symptoms are not due to estrogen loss, but are simply a result of hot flashes and lack of adequate sleep."

When you realize that more than 300 types of tissues throughout the body have receptors for estrogen—which is to say that they're affected in some way by the hormone—it is not surprising that its decrease would cause physical changes.

"Estrogen affects the genital organs (vagina, vulva and uterus), the urinary organs (bladder and urethra), breasts, skin, hair, mucous membranes, bones, heart and blood vessels, pelvic muscles and the brain," Giller continues. "It's the loss of estrogen to these organs that causes the ultimate changes of menopause, including dry hair and skin, incontinence and susceptibility to urinary tract infections, vaginal dryness, and, most important, the diseases osteoporosis and heart disease. These diseases are at the center of the controversy concerning menopause. Because estrogen plays a role in preventing these diseases, should you replace the estrogen lost at the time of menopause with a synthetic version?"

Change of life is a very specific thing for a woman—the end of her monthly cycle, explained Richard A. Kunin, M.D., in *Mega-Nutrition for Women*. But it also has overt metabolic consequences, such as the infamous "hot flashes" and other mild discomforts. This time of life signals the approach of "old age" and associated feelings of sexual decline and perhaps depression.

However, a great deal of psychological reaction colors our understanding of menopause. Irritability and mood swings are often attributed to a woman's undergoing the one-to-two-year period of change of life, when perhaps all we really see are the discomfort and embarrassment of flushes, sometimes the insomnia and fatigue that result from those flushes when they occur throughout the night.

"Psychiatric illness is now known to be no more common at the menopausal age—about 48 to 52, with a trend upward—than at other times," Kunin said. "Dr. Myrna Weissman of the Yale University School of Medicine confirmed this in a study of depression and precipitating stresses among women between ages of 45 and 55 and younger and older groups. Other research indicates only a slight increase in requests for psychiatric treatment at the menopausal age. Life stresses that are common in this period can be considered 'midlife crises,' and are similar for men and women: the maturation of the family, the diminution of enthusiasm for one's job, the questioning of one's sexual powers. But women suffer other, more specific problems directly related to hormonal changes, such as urinary tract infections, difficulty of sexual intercourse and probably a tendency to obesity."

Our understanding and treatment of these problems, as well as of the problems of aging in general, are keyed in an obvious way to nutrition and nutrient therapy, since the brain is the major factor in how we react to hormonal changes and in how those changes can be affected. And as we learn more about that marvelous supercomputer that regulates every function of our body, we are beginning to find that drugs and medications are the enemy and that only through the body's own biochemicals can we hope to improve our brain functioning and thus our quality of life.

The first sign that menopause is approaching is usually abnormal menstrual bleeding, ranging from skipping just one period to intramenstrual spotting, to a sudden cessation of menstruation for several months or permanently, according to Niels Laurensen, M.D., and Steven Whitney in *A Woman's Body*. This pattern can persist for several years, depending on the individual's estrogen level. Irregular menstruation can, however, be a sign of several conditions and a woman who experiences those symptoms should see a gynecologist to have the bleeding abnormality evaluated and her estrogen level checked. This is especially true for middle-aged women who experience a resumption of vaginal bleeding after more than a six-month cessation of menstruation. This might be an early sign of uterine cancer.

Only 25 percent of American women suffer any significant menopausal symptoms, other than cessation of ovulation and menstruation. The most severe and abrupt changes occur in women who have undergone surgically induced menopause via hysterectomy and oopherectomy (removal of ovaries). These women suffer from two types of symptoms. One type is due to vascular instability (hot flashes, sweating, etc.). The second type is thought to be primarily psychosomatic, and are generally consistent with what a woman has been told about menopause—heart pain, hysteria, constipation, ulcers and depression.

"To the extent that they are physical, menopausal symptoms are probably due to low levels of estrogen and high levels of gonadotrophins—FSH and LH," Laurensen and Whitney say. "These hormonal changes affect the brain, and it should be understood that although many symptoms may be psychosomatic, they are grounded in physiological imbalance."

Writing in *Natural Health, Natural Medicine,* Andrew Weil, M.D., stated that "Many women sail through the change of life with minimal discomfort, and I see many vital postmenopausal women who have never taken replacement hormones. Mental attitude has a lot to do with how you experience menopause. If you see it as a tragic end to youth and sexuality, it will cause you great distress and leave you susceptible to the persuasions of those who will try to sell you eternal youth in the form of pills. If you see it as a natural transition to the next phase of life, you can accept it with serenity and without the help of the medical profession."

One of the things that regular menstrual periods do is to flush toxins out of the body, according to Carolyn Dean, M.D., in *Dr. Carolyn Dean's Complementary Natural Prescriptions for Common Ailments.* And she wonders if the cessation of regular bleeding is one reason why more women develop arthritic symptoms during menopause. She believes these women are holding onto more toxins, which can then be deposited in the joint spaces. For that reason, she recommends that women in the menopausal years should start some form of detoxification. In Japan and other countries, women do not seem to experience the same symptoms of menopause that women do in North America. There is very little hot flushing, depression or mood change in this normal phase of a woman's life. Therefore, all of these symptoms can be regarded as either dietary, psychological or psychosocial.

Menopause has come to be regarded by most medical practitioners as a disease process rather than as an evolutionary life transition, according to Farida Sharan, M.D.M.A., M.H., in the April/May 1995 issue of *Alternative and Complementary Therapies.* Therefore, primary care doctors must create a respectful context to approach each woman's experience before treating her menopause. Physical, emotional, sexual and mental influences of menopause create a uniquely personal transition, which must be supported with the greatest consideration by the practitioner.

Natural treatment does not treat isolated symptoms separately from constitutional aging, lifestyle influences, the state of health at the start of menopause, emotional recovery and the development of chronic disease. Symptoms are also influenced by a woman's past and present stress, levels of exhaustion and depletion, dietary habits, the function of the eliminative systems, and expectations and attitude toward the change of life.

"Health care professionals need to inspire women to work actively and creatively with their menopause and to overcome the challenges that may occur in any area or dimension of their lives," Sharan said. "Especially during this time, clinicians cannot separate physical symptoms from the emerging dynamics of emotional recovery. During a consultation, the practitioner must consider all areas or aspects of a woman's life that may be denied, frustrated, blocked or unborn. Women must be educated to cooperate with the healing processes of purification, regeneration and transformation as they undergo treatment for menopause."

As a woman enters her forties and begins the aging process, she often experiences symptoms, disease crises and emotional imbalances, Sharan continued. Emotions can become excessive as a woman gets in touch with deeper levels of herself. She also becomes more aware of relationships and life situations that may need to change. A woman may experience rage, depression, grief, fear and loss as she seeks resolution of various issues. Menopause, therefore, is a time for a woman to take time for herself, to nourish herself, to explore her being and to become more deeply involved with her own life process.

Sharan added that traditional approaches to menopause include the use of prescriptive hormones. But, while these medications offer welcome support, they are not a substitute for the inner work of each individual woman as she progresses on her life journey. Although these treatments are administered with the best of intentions and may relieve the present situation, deeper life processes are not usually considered.

"It is the responsibility of all physicians to inspire and support women to work consciously with their midlife transition," Sharan maintained. "When a woman receives love, support, understanding and respect for her personal process, growth and healing are encouraged and nourished at the deepest levels. As this happens on an expanded scale, health care professionals create resources for supporting menopause as a birthing into the wisdom years. This change of attitude will inspire women to prepare for, and participate in, the change of life with enthusiasm, joy, courage and self-love."

"Do not add avoidable difficulties to those that may occur naturally during the years of menopause," advises *The American Medical Association Family Medical Guide*. "For example, do not neglect your health or personal appearance. If you have a lot of leisure time, especially if you have children who are no longer living at home, develop new interests and friends."

If you wish to avoid pregnancy during this time, the guide continues, you should know that the possible period of fertility depends on your age at the time of your last period. If you are under 50, you should continue to use contraceptives for 24 months after the date of your last period. If you are over 50, you should protect yourself for 12 months after the last period.

"If you are having hot flashes and sweating," the guide added, "remember that usually you will be the only person who is aware of them. If sweating is a nuisance at night, wear absorbent cotton night clothes. If you find that intercourse makes your vagina sore, use a lubricant such as a water-soluble jelly."

Some women undergoing menopause experience sudden and severe hot flashes, their vaginal walls may become thinner and lose moisture, and intercourse may cause bleeding and pain, according to James Marti and Andrea Hine in *The Alternative Health and Medicine Encyclopedia*. Vaginal itching and burning can occur, and women are more susceptible to yeast and bacterial infections, due to menopausal hormone changes that disrupt the delicate pH of the vagina. In addition, menopause can be accompanied by a loss of muscle tone in the pelvic region, resulting in stress incontinence (urine leakage when coughing, laughing or exercising vigorously), and a drop of pelvic organs. As estrogen production declines, the relative increase in testosterone (also produced in the ovaries) may result in the growth of facial hair and thinning of scalp hair.

"The National Institute of Aging warns in *The Menopausal Time of Life* that mood changes may occur during menopause," say Marti and Hine. "Other common symptoms include fatigue, nervousness, excess sweating, breathlessness, headaches, sleeplessness, joint pain, depression, irritability and impatience. These symptoms may be due to shifting hormonal balances or other factors such as heredity, general health, nutrition, medications, exercise, stressful life events (such as grown children leaving home or the need to care for parents who are ill) and attitude. The Institute counsels women to develop a positive attitude toward menopause, regarding it as a normal life change (instead of as the end of a useful life) and continuing to participate in satisfying activities."

A study reported by Greg Glutfeld in the March 1993 issue of *Prevention*, the authors continued, suggests that slow, deep breathing can relieve some of the symptoms of menopause, including hot flashes. A group of women experiencing frequent hot flashes practiced one of three options: slow, deep breathing, muscle relaxation or brainwave (EEG) biofeedback. Muscle relaxation and biofeedback had no effect, while deep breathing was linked to 50 percent fewer hot flashes. Slow, deep abdominal breathing probably reduces hot flashes by diminishing the arousal of the central nervous system that normally occurs in the initiation of hot flashes. This technique may be useful for women with hot flashes who cannot receive hormone replacement therapy due to other health reasons.

HOT FLASHES

Reddening of the face, neck and upper trunk is usually facilitated by decreased estrogen hormone production by the ovaries during or after the menopause, explained Charles B. Clayman, M.D., in *The American Medical Association Home Medical Encyclopedia*. A hot flash typically lasts one to two minutes and is accompanied by a sensation of heat. And it is often followed by sweating. Hot flashes are aggravated when the sufferer is under stress.

"Hot flashes may also occur after a total hysterectomy, in which the uterus and the ovaries are removed," Clayman says. "Occasionally, men experience hot flashes after orchiectomy (removal of a testis), which causes a reduction in testosterone levels. If hot flashes are severe, they can usually be alleviated by hormone replacement therapy."

Hot flashes and night sweats are experienced by up to 85 percent of all woman, according to *The Physicians' Manual for Patients*. Although the mechanism of these symptoms is not yet understood, they seem to result from a vasomotor (the body's temperature regulation system) instability related to changing hormonal levels.

The hallmark of hot flashes is a sudden suffusion of heat affecting the face and upper part of the body. There may be a red blotching of the skin and excessive perspiration, followed by a chill. Their frequency and intensity varies considerably among women, ranging from the barely noticeable to the almost intolerable. Fortunately, the body almost always adjusts to the decreased levels of female hormones, and the flushes lessen and disappear.

"The hot flashes usually occur without warning and may be over in a moment or may last for as long as a minute," the manual says. "Although many women experience discomfort from these flashes and are embarrassed because they fear they are obvious to those around them, the latter usually is not the case. Night sweats, another term for hot flashes that occur during sleep, are sometimes severe enough to disrupt sleep and, consequently, may give rise to the increased irritability, fatigue or feelings of depression often associated with menopause. It should be emphasized that mood changes are not menopausal symptoms per se but instead may be consequences of concurrent factors in the woman's life, such as feeling unneeded as children move on their own or as career and other roles change."

If you take your temperature during an episode of hot flashes, you may find that you don't have any real fever, reported Howard R. and Martha E. Lewis in *The People's Medical Manual*. These hot flashes may start from two to five years before the actual menopause, and may continue for several years thereafter. They can occur during the day or night. Some women experience as many as 20 or more a day, and may be awakened by this sensation several times a night. Other women are barely troubled.

Hot flashes are thought to be caused by the sudden excessive dilation (expanding) of small blood vessels close to the skin's surface. This results in more blood being brought to the area, which produces increased local heat and activates the sweat glands. As previously mentioned, the instability of the blood vessels that cause the flashes is probably due to changes in hormone production.

"Other common symptoms associated with menopause are dizziness, weakness, insomnia, nervousness, headache and backache," the Lewises note. "There may be sharp changes in blood pressure, heart palpitations or stomach upsets. There may also be weight gain or redistribution of weight, and breast pains. Brown patches may develop, especially in areas exposed to light, such as in the face, hands, arms or legs. A woman may also experience a recurrence of skin allergy."

During hot flashes, the face and upper body—sometimes the entire body—become very warm and flushed as skin temperature suddenly rises 7° to 8° F. Hot flashes usually stop in the two to nine years it takes the body to get used to a lack of estrogen, they said.

Sadja Greenwood, M.D., observes in *Menopause, Naturally*: "The popular image of the middle-aged woman as an emotional wreck, drenched in sweat and unable to cope, has been played up by pharmaceutical companies to persuade doctors and their patients to use drugs for this condition."

It seems preferable to try to avoid anything that raises body temperature, such as alcohol, caffeine, hot drinks, hot meals, warm rooms and emotional upsets. And avoid smoking, since smoke reduces the amount of estrogen your body manufactures.

Greenwood suggests that women prone to hot flashes should keep cool. If possible, open a bedroom window at night when hot flashes and related sweats keep you from getting the rest you need. One reason that menopausal women seem to be tired or to have difficulty concentrating is that hot flashes keep them from getting enough sleep. Wear layers of clothes that you can easily peel off when a hot flash begins, eat frequent small meals, maintain your normal weight and drink iced water or juice after exercise.

Robert M. Giller, M.D. noted in *Natural Prescriptions* that drops in blood sugar can be the single most common precipitating cause of hot flashes. Once the blood sugar is controlled, the incidence of hot flashes diminishes. In fact, many women have told him that their hot flashes were dramatically relieved by following the suggestions concerning hypoglycemia (low blood sugar) in his book, particularly eliminating sugar, reducing caffeine, eating meals at regular times, eating protein at lunch and dinner, and taking the supplement chromium.

Hot flashes can be treated by making sure the adrenal glands are supported in their production of female hormones as they take over from the ovaries, according to Carolyn Dean, M.D. in *Dr. Carolyn Dean's Complementary Natural Prescriptions for*

Common Ailments. And, she notes, hot flashes occur less in women who have regular intercourse—at least once a week.

"If the adrenal glands are exhausted," she said, "it might be more difficult for this hormone production to occur and support must be given in the form of desiccated adrenal, one or two tablets twice a day, mid-morning and mid-afternoon; pantothenic acid, a B vitamin that supports the adrenal glands, 500 mg three times a day; vitamin C, which supports the adrenal glands, 1,000 mg two times a day; vitamin E, 400 I.U., one or two per day will aid the circulation and the liver. Ginseng as well as black cohosh can be useful herbs."

There is a rich folklore about what triggers hot flashes, with external factors such as stress, caffeine, spicy foods and even sexual intercourse named as culprits, explained Bernadine Healy, M.D., in *A New Prescription for Women's Health*. The truth is, she said, that most hot flashes are unpredictable. Only two factors have been definitely shown to increase the severity of hot flashes: smoking, which aggravates all early menopausal symptoms, and hysterectomy with ovary removal.

"Many studies have shown," she said, "that women in other cultures may not experience hot flashes. In some Asian societies, such as Japan, there is not even a word for this symptom. A recent report showed that Mayan women who underwent menopause had the same hormonal profile of decreased estrogen and increased follicle-stimulating hormone as other women who had menopausal symptoms, but these women did not report hot flashes. Perhaps some of these cultures simply preclude women from reporting health difficulties they are indeed undergoing, but I suspect we may someday find a valuable lesson in whatever biological, cultural or nutritional origins account for these different experiences. Soybeans, for example, are high in plant estrogens, and are perhaps mitigating menopausal symptoms in Japanese women, who have diets rich in soy products such as tofu."

This theory was explored in more detail by Herman Adlercreutz and Esa Hamalainen in *The Lancet* in 1992. They reported that high levels of isoflavonoid phytoestrogens—in such products as tofu, miso, aburage, atuage, koridofu, soybeans and boiled beans—may partly explain why hot flashes and other menopausal symptoms are reduced in Japanese women.

VAGINAL DRYNESS

Another symptom directly related to the hormonal changes of menopause is vaginal dryness, according to *The Physicians' Manual for Patients*. This condition, which often leads to itching, infection and discomfort during sexual intercourse, is relieved by the use of lubricating cream. Since many women experience a strong resurgence of sexual desire at menopause, problems in this area should be frankly discussed with your doctor so that they can be resolved promptly.

Late in the menopausal period, vaginal tissues may become thin and shrunken. These tissues lose their elasticity and become dry and easily irritated. Known as atrophic vaginitis, this condition can make sexual intercourse painful. A water-soluble jelly such as K-Y can be used as a lubricant. Treatment with estrogen creams can relieve the problem, but they are absorbed into the body and may be no safer than estrogen taken orally.

"Vaginal dryness can make sexual intercourse difficult, but it does not mean that your sex life is at an end," according to Andrew Weil, M.D., in *Natural Health, Natural Medicine*. "Try . . . an over-the-counter vaginal lotion and get in the habit of using lubricant jellies before sex. If these fail to help, your doctor can prescribe a topical estrogen cream and instruct you in its use. Used occasionally, this will restore normal vaginal tissue, and although some of the estrogen cream will be systematically absorbed, it will be a fraction of what you would get with estrogen replacement."

A dry vagina is usually another side effect of lowered estrogen levels at menopause, although psychological factors may also be a factor, reported Ellen Michaud, Lila L. Anastas, et al., in *Listen to Your Body*.

They reported that Michael R. Spence, M.D. said that, "A lot of women won't lubricate adequately to intercourse. One of the reasons is inadequate stimulation or plain old boredom. Another is inadequate foreplay. One more is friction in the family."

Spence went on, "Let's say, for example, that a woman found out that her husband's been seeing someone else. They can foreplay until the cows come home and she just isn't going to lubricate. So when I talk to a woman who says she isn't lubricating adequately, we spend a fair amount of time talking about the relationship between her and her sexual partner. He may have seen someone several months ago, and she may think 'We're over that now,' but she's really not. And we need to take some time with that."

"Another way to prevent a dry vagina, researchers say, is to keep sexually active," the authors continued. "In a study of 54 women over age 60, the famous research team, Masters and Johnson, found that the three women in the study who remained sexually active throughout menopause were the only women who responded to sexual stimulation with a flood of vaginal lubrication."

A study of 52 postmenopausal women at the New Jersey-Rutgers Medical School revealed that women aged 50 through 65 who had intercourse three or more times a month did not experience the vaginal shrinkage of menopause that usually accompanies dryness.

Painful intercourse can be related to a pelvic inflammatory disease or endometriosis; a vaginal infection; a prolapsed or tipped uterus; ovarian cysts; vestibular adenitis, an inflammation of the mucus-producing gland near the entrance of the vagina; vaginismus, which causes vaginal muscle spasms; cervical polyps; a dry vagina due to menopause; tumors or pelvic adhesions, the authors said. Anticipating the pain may prevent vaginal lubrication and compound the problem.

Spence advises that, if you've had comfortable intercourse for many years and then all of a sudden it becomes painful, you should be checked by a gynecologist. You may simply need a temporary hormone supplement or vaginal lubrication or, if infection is causing the pain, an antibiotic. Or maybe you just need to change positions when you have intercourse. A tipped uterus can be painful when it's hit by a thrusting penis. However, if you flip over and have intercourse on your hands and knees or on your back with a big pillow under your bottom, the uterus "tips" back into a less painful position. If painful intercourse continues despite treatment or a change of positions, your doctor may suggest surgery.

"But pain caused by an involuntary tightening of your vaginal muscles—one that may even make penetration impossible—may respond to 'retraining,'" according to *Listen to Your Body*. "One way, experts suggest, is to insert one finger at a time into the vagina until you can insert several fingers. If you do this exercise daily, intercourse with pleasure—and not pain—may well be your just reward."

OSTEOPOROSIS

Osteoporosis (porous bone) is a disorder of the bone in which excessive loss of bone tissue results in decreased bone mineral density and increased susceptibility to fracture. An estimated 25 million Americans—80 percent of them women—are affected by this condition. It is estimated that osteoporosis accounts for about 1.5 million fractures each year, including 500,000 vertebral fractures, over 250,000 hip fractures and

200,000 wrist fractures. It is estimated that about 70 percent of the fractures occurring in people over the age of 45 are a result of osteoporosis-related complications.

Although it is difficult to pinpoint the exact cause of osteoporosis, the disorder occurs when there is a shift of the lifelong process of bone formation and bone loss, where bone loss exceeds bone formation. And the drop in estrogen levels when women reach menopause seems to play a significant role in this process. In addition to fractures, common warning signs of osteoporosis are chronic aching of the spine or back, loss of height and development of curvature in the upper back (dowager's hump).

Risk factors for osteoporosis include: 1) Being female; 2) advanced age; 3) being underweight and having a small body frame; 4) being Caucasian or Asian, although African-Americans and Hispanics are also at risk: 5) early menopause; 6) chronically low calcium and vitamin D intake; 7) lack of physical activity; 8) history of smoking; 9) excessive alcohol and/or caffeine intake; and 10) family history of the disease.

Smoking, which seems to attract many older women, is related to many health problems other than osteoporosis. In fact, smoking is a risk to early menopause, according to Andre S. Midgette and John A. Baron, of the Dartmouth Medical School in the November 1990 issue of *Epidemiology*. They found that smokers had almost double the risk of menopause between the ages of 44 and 55. However, those who had quit smoking had a lowered risk, suggesting there could be a partial reversal of the effect.

Matti J. Valimaki, M.D., and colleagues at the Cardiovascular Risk in Young Finns Study Group, reported in the *British Medical Journal* in 1994 that exercising regularly and abstaining from smoking during the teen-age years may help to ward off osteoporosis later in life.

After a woman reaches menopause, bone density usually drops about one percent a year, stated Gustawa Stendig-Lindberg, M.D., of the Tel Aviv University Sackler School of Medicine in the July 22, 1993 issue of *Medical Tribune*. It is believed that magnesium may halt the loss of bone because of its importance in the transport of calcium in and out of the cells.

During the childbearing years, a woman needs a strong skeleton and a healthy reserve of calcium in case she becomes pregnant and later nurses children. After menopause, she no longer has the same need for this protective reserve of calcium. As her estrogen level drops, her bones start to contribute a larger share of calcium to meet the body's needs. And some scientists believe that a chronic shortage in dietary calcium is one important factor leading to osteoporosis.

If daily calcium losses are not balanced by adequate amounts of calcium in the diet, the bones begin to break down to maintain the proper blood level of calcium.

Other causes of bone loss include: 1) Medications such as corticosteroids (to treat arthritis and other diseases) and heparin (an anticoagulant); 2) diseases such as hyperthyroidism, hyperparathyroidism, kidney disease and certain forms of cancer (lymphoma, leukemia and multiple myeloma); 3) impaired ability to absorb calcium from the intestine, caused by diseases of the small intestine, liver or pancreas; and 4) excessive excretion of calcium in the urine.

"Although no one knows exactly what causes osteoporosis, the rapid acceleration of the condition after menopause suggests a strong hormonal link," reported *Family Physicians Care for America Media Update,* for Fall 1987. "Consequently, after the onset of menopause—whether natural or surgically induced through removal of the ovaries—estrogen replacement therapy is frequently recommended." Estrogen replacement has a significant effect in preventing osteoporosis, but, to be most effective, it must be started as soon as possible after menopause. (The pros and cons of ERT are discussed elsewhere in this book.)

Other deterrents to osteoporosis include calcitonin—a hormone secreted by the thyroid gland that regulates the level of calcium in the blood and stimulates bone production—and fluoride, both of which are still being studied, and calcium supplements.

HEART DISEASE

Next to osteoporosis, the biggest health threat that overtakes menopausal women is heart disease. One of the most interesting reports in this area came in a 1978 update of the Framingham Study. That study, begun in 1948, involved the residents of Framingham, Massachusetts, when 5,209 people were enrolled, given a thorough heart examination and invited to return every two years for new evaluations.

By 1978, most of the women in the study had ceased menstruating. Not one of the 2,873 women in the study had a heart attack or died of heart disease before menopause. After menopause, heart disease was common. For women aged 45 to 54, the incidence of heart disease during or after menopause was double the rate before menopause.

It is significant that there is a big jump in cholesterol in the blood at menopause, mostly due to a rise in low-density lipoprotein cholesterol (LDL), the kind that is especially associated with heart disease. Japanese researchers have also found higher levels of triglycerides, another fat that is implicated in heart disease, in the blood of postmenopausal women.

Researchers say that good nutrition can help to prevent heart disease after menopause. Garlic is one nutrient that can contribute to blood vessel and heart health, and the use of garlic extract products allows the intake of more therapeutic quantities of the active ingredients than even a fairly adventurous diet would provide. And women who smoke have a greater chance of developing heart disease.

INSOMNIA

During menopause there is atrophy of estrogen-dependent tissues, such as breast tissue and the vaginal lining, and sleep becomes more fragmented, with awakenings often related to hot flashes or night sweats.

Menstrual-associated sleep disorder, a disorder of unknown cause, is characterized by insomnia or excessive sleepiness related to the menses or menopause. It exists in three forms: insomnia or hypersomnia (abnormally deep or prolonged sleep) related to the menstrual cycle, and insomnia which occurs during menopause.

Sleeping pills are to be avoided for dealing with insomnia associated with menopause, or, indeed, with any other cause. Relaxation techniques can be useful, as can some traditional herbal remedies. Preparations available from herbalists or health stores containing valerian, chamomile or hops can be effective in many cases of insomnia.

HEADACHES

Researchers are still unraveling the various causes of headaches. They range from allergies, sinusitis, eyestrain and sex to hunger and hypoglycemia. Headaches are a side effect of menopause, although migraines are often reduced after menopause because estrogen levels are consistently low.

Migraine headaches often involve a hereditary predisposition. For those with this predisposition, stress can cause constriction of the brain's arteries (the pre-headache phase). This is followed by a sudden dilation or opening up of the portions of these arteries (the headache phase). The dilation stretches the nerve endings that encircle the arteries, resulting in pain.

Migraine headaches often stop after menopause because there is less fluctuation in the secretion of female hormones in the body: in other words, no hormones, no headaches, reported Seymour Diamond, M.D., in *The Hormone Headache*.

He discussed a 55-year-old patient, who had had migraine attacks for 40 years. Menopause had come and gone, but the migraines persisted and were bothering her at the rate of two or three a week. Diamond soon learned that she had begun taking female hormone pills when she passed through menopause.

"She refused to give up the hormone pills because she feared a loss of feminity and osteoporosis," Diamond said. "For years she had heard of the dangers of osteoporosis and the propensity for hip fractures in women who did not remain on hormone supplements. Despite the fact that I suggested that the hormone tablets might be the cause of her problem, she just couldn't or wouldn't stop taking them."

Later, after complaining of a migraine, she also developed a paralysis of her right arm and right leg and was convinced that she had had a stroke. After admitting her to the hospital, Diamond determined that she had not had a stroke but had a severe episode of complicated, or hemiplegic, migraine. It is often difficult to distinguish between this and a stroke in older patients, he added.

"Soon we were sure that my diagnosis was correct," says Diamond. "We treated [her], not for stroke but for complicated migraine. She recovered from her paralysis quickly. The migraine, being deeply involved with the blood vessels around the brain, had merely caused a complication that mimicked the appearance of a stroke. The incident had given her a good scare, though, enough so that I was able to get her off the hormone pills. Within a matter of weeks, her severe headaches dissipated, and now she suffers from only an occasional, very mild migraine."

Another patient, a 48-year-old woman who was taking hormone replacement therapy, complained of severe migraines one hour after rigorous aerobic exercise. A nine-hour migraine attack, complete with dizziness, sent her to her doctor and to a neurologist, who told her that the headaches had begun after she had switched from oral estrogen replacement pills to the estrogen patch she wore constantly on her buttocks.

"The mystery of the post-exercise headaches was solved. When the woman attended her aerobics classes it boosted her blood circulation and increased her absorption of estrogen from the patch on her buttocks. The additional estrogen then triggered a severe headache. When the woman later took off her estrogen patch during her aerobics classes, she had no further headaches."

Headache remedies, prescription or over-the-counter, are a dubious proposition, with some studies indicating that half of chronic headaches are actually *caused* by the drugs intended to prevent or cure them. Homeopathic and herbal remedies have a good reputation for effectiveness and safety, and British studies reported in *The Lancet* have demonstrated a remarkable curative effect on usually intractable migraines with the herb feverfew.

THE PROS AND CONS OF ESTROGEN REPLACEMENT THERAPY

Since Mother Nature in her infinite wisdom gradually shuts down the production of estrogen as a woman enters menopause, the logical question is: why should synthetic estrogen then be introduced into the woman's body, since she is no longer able to have children? This debate has been going on for years, and it is likely to continue for many more.

Holistic physicians often prescribe estrogen replacement therapy (ERT) for various conditions, especially for young women who have had a hysterectomy, but they prefer more natural procedures. On the other hand, their allopathic counterparts seem to recommend ERT as easily as they prescribe aspirin. Women who are facing a hysterectomy—especially young women—should get a second, third or even fourth opinion from an alternative medicine practitioner. A hysterectomy is somewhat analogous to a male having his testicles surgically removed, leaving emotional scars that can last a lifetime. Therefore, this procedure should be weighed carefully before allowing it to happen.

The treatment of menopause-related symptoms is complicated. Estrogen replacement therapy usually alleviates most symptoms of menopause and may prevent some of its long-term complications, such as osteoporosis and coronary heart disease. A number of studies have suggested that taking postmenopausal estrogen reduces the risk of hip fractures by about 50 percent. Studies have also shown that estrogen reduces the risk of coronary heart disease and cardiovascular death in women by as much as 50 percent.

But hormone replacement therapy does have side effects. Many studies indicate that taking estrogen by itself is associated with increased risk of endometrial cancer. Yearly monitoring with an endometrial biopsy, a procedure that can be done in a physician's office, or combining a progesterone hormone with estrogen therapy can reduce this risk.

Regardless of the choice of hormone therapy, most women who are receiving hormone replacement and have not had a prior hysterectomy will have some vaginal bleeding. A relationship between long-term estrogen therapy and cancer of the breast has been speculated but not proved. Furthermore, there are women, such as those who previously have had cancers of the breast or uterus, for whom estrogen therapy is contraindicated. And for women who have other conditions—gallstones, migraine headaches, etc.—estrogen therapy may have other risks.

The American College of Physicians recommends that all postmenopausal women be considered candidates for hormone therapy but that before starting estrogen replacement every woman discuss the specific benefits and risks with her doctor.

Estrogen therapy after menopause will protect women's bones only if they continue treatment for seven to 10 years, stated Saralie Faivelson in the November 4, 1993 issue of *Medical Tribune*.

David T. Felson, M.D., of the Boston University School of Medicine, who conducted the study, was quoted as saying that if treatment is stopped years before a woman turns 75, no protective effect will remain. He added that, "Elderly women, who are at the highest risk of osteoporotic fracture, have no residual protective effect on their bones from the estrogen they took around the time of menopause."

The largest study of its kind ever conducted has found that women who take estrogen after menopause run an increased risk of developing breast cancer, reported Gina Kolata in the November 28, 1990 issue of *The New York Times*. But, she said, experts said the findings did not mean that postmenopausal women should stop taking estrogen. They said that the benefits of the drug are great and the increased risk of breast cancer is relatively small.

Many researchers are highly suspicious of estrogen because the idea that it causes cancer fits into their notion of how breast cancer grows. Epidemiologists have noted that almost anything that increases a woman's exposure to estrogen increases her chances of getting breast cancer. The younger a girl is when she starts to menstruate, the greater her chances of developing breast cancer when she is older. And the older a woman is when she stops menstruating, the greater her likelihood of developing breast cancer.

Biologists have found that estrogen stimulates the growth of breast tissue. Many breast cancer cells are actually fueled by estrogen. The cancer cells have proteins protruding from them that latch onto estrogen and use the hormone to stimulate their growth.

Women who take estrogen for 10 years or more are twice as likely to develop asthma as women who have never taken the hormone, according to Denise Mann in the December 21, 1995 issue of *Medical Tribune*. The study's author, Frank E. Speizer, M.D., of the Harvard Medical School in Boston, said that in a study of over 90,000 women, past or current estrogen use increased the risk of asthma by about 50 percent.

Writing in *Dr. Whitaker's Guide to Natural Healing*, Julian Whitaker, M.D. said that the healthy diet and lifestyle choices he outlined in his book are, in his opinion, the best ways to prevent the chronic problems often associated with menopause. These changes alone have been shown to provide some of the same beneficial effects of estrogen replacement therapy, without the risks. They are also the best way to maintain vitality during the aging process. But, he said, despite their value, these natural treatments are recommended less often than hormone replacement therapy.

Side effects of estrogen therapy include: increased risk of cancer, increased risk of gallstones, increased risk for stroke or heart attack, nausea, symptoms similar to PMS, breast tenderness, depression, liver disorders, enlargement of uterine fibroids, fluid retention, blood sugar disturbances and headache.

"Many chronic conditions are associated with long-term administration of estrogen," Whitaker continued. "Women show an increased risk of developing certain cancers, principally breast cancer. But a drug like estrogen, which must be administered from age 50 until death at 70, 80, or 90, is an extremely profitable product. A pharmaceutical firm wants science to say that the drug is valuable, because once a patient is on them, it is usually for life."[5]

In an in-depth review of estrogen in the June 26, 1995 issue of *Time*, Claudia Wallis wrote that, "Estrogen is indeed the closest thing in modern medicine to an elixir of youth—

a drug that slows the ravages of time for women. It is already the No. 1 prescription drug in America, and it is about to hit its demographic sweet spot: the millions of baby boomers now experiencing their first hot flashes. What Robert A. Wilson, M.D. [an earlier proponent of estrogen] didn't appreciate, but what today's women should know, is that, like every other magic potion, this one has a dark side. To gain the full benefits of estrogen, a woman must take it not only at menopause but also for decades afterward. It means a lifetime of drug taking and possible side effects that include an increased risk of several forms of cancer. That danger was underscored last week by a report in *The New England Journal of Medicine* reaffirming the long-suspected link between estrogen-replacement therapy and breast cancer. Weighing such risks against the truly marvelous benefits of estrogen may be the most difficult health decision a woman can make. And there's no avoiding it."

For many women, Wallis continued, there is something fundamentally disturbing about turning a normal event like menopause into a disease that demands decades of medication. And there's something spooky about continuing to have monthly bleeding at age 60, a fairly common consequence of some types of hormone therapy. She quoted Dr. Nada Stotland, 51, an HRT dropout and a psychiatrist at the University of Chicago, who said, "Why fight vainly to remain in a stage of life you can't be in any more, instead of enjoying the stage you are in?" Stotland is "extra skeptical because there are powerful forces that aim one toward prescribed hormones, but there is no profit motive in not prescribing something."

Isaac Schiff, M.D., chief of obstetrics and gynecology at Massachusetts General Hospital, expressed his skepticism in another way: "Basically, you're presenting women with the possibility of increasing the risk of getting breast cancer at age 60 in order to prevent a heart attack at age 70 and a hip fracture at age 80. How can you make that decision for a patient?"

It remains for each woman to weigh the risks and to decide for herself whether or not she wants to take estrogen replacement therapy.

BLACK COHOSH FOR MENOPAUSE

Black cohosh (*Cimicifuga racemosa (L.) Nutt.*) was widely used by American Indians and later by American colonists for the relief of menstrual cramps and menopause, according to Melvyn R. Werbach, M.D. and Michael T. Murray, N.D. in *Botanical Influences on Illness*. This was due to the herb's estrogenic effects.

They reviewed an experimental study, originally published in *Planta Medica*, in which 110 menopausal women were given either 8 mg/day of an ethanolic extract of the rhizome (rootlike underground form) of black cohosh (Remifemin) or a placebo. After eight weeks of therapy, luteinizing hormone (LH), but not follicle-stimulating hormone (FSH), levels were significantly reduced in the women given the black cohosh extract, suggesting a significant estrogenic effect. In an animal study, the researchers concluded that the black cohosh extracts resulted in the LH-suppressive effect due to at least three synergistically acting compounds.

The herb, a member of the Ranunculaceae or buttercup family, is also known as black snakeroot, bugbane and squawroot. It is a stately perennial, three to eight feet tall, that is topped by a long plume of white flowers when it blooms from June through September. In North America, it is found from Ontario south to Georgia and Tennessee, and from Massachusetts west to Missouri. Since the plant has prominent white flowers, you might expect it to be called white cohosh. But the "black" in its name refers to the dark color of the rhizome. The strong odor of the plant's flowers acts as an insect repellent, hence the name "bugbane." *Cimicifuga* in Latin means "bug repellent."

A brew made from the rhizome was a favored Indian remedy for menstrual cramps and the pains of childbirth, hence the name "squawroot." Indians also used a poultice made from the rhizome for a snakebite.

In the 19th century, a tincture made from the rhizome was deemed helpful for treating rheumatism. Laboratory experiments suggest that extracts of the rhizome have an antiinflammatory effect and that its use in the treatment of neralgia and rheumatism may therefore be well founded.

Sometimes referred to as black snakeroot or cimicifuga, the dried rhizome and roots of black cohosh have an ancient reputation as a remedy for the treatment of all kinds of "female complaints," reported Varro E. Tyler, Ph.D., Sc.D., in *Herbs of Choice: The Therapeutic Use of Phytomedicinals.* "R. Hansel has reviewed the literature supporting claims of estrogen-like activity for extracts of black cohosh," Tyler said. "A clinical study of hysterectomized patients with climacteric symptoms showed no significant differences among groups treated with various estrogens and those with black cohosh extracts. The beneficial effects were slow to appear, requiring up to four weeks to reach a maximum. More recently, however, investigators have shown that an alcoholic extract of black cohosh suppressed hot flashes in menopausal women by reducing the secretion of luteinizing hormone. It also suppressed LH production in ovariectomized rats."

Tyler went on to say that a German government commission found black cohosh to be effective for the treatment of premenstrual syndrome and dysmenorrhea, as well as nervous conditions associated with menopause. The herb is normally administered in the form of a 40 to 60 percent alcoholic extract in a quantity equivalent to 40 mg of drug daily standardized for 1 mg of 27-deoxyactein. A decoction prepared from 0.3 to 2.0 g of the herb may also be employed. Administration of the drug sometimes causes stomach upsets; otherwise, no problems or contraindications have been reported. Tyler suggested that administration of the herb should be limited to a period of no longer than six months without direct medical supervision.

Clinical findings have shown that black cohosh promotes and/or restores healthy menstrual activity, soothes irritation and congestion of the uterus, cervix and vagina, relieves the pain and distress of pregnancy, contributes to quick, easy and uncomplicated deliveries, and promotes uterine involution and recovery. In support of the clinical findings, research has found hypotensive principles, vasodilatory, estrogenic, anti-inflammatory and uterine contractile activity. Although the exact mode of action remains a mystery, black cohosh appears to act both directly on the tissues of the reproductive system and indirectly through the nervous system. The plant is a primary nerve and smooth muscle relaxant.

Black cohosh has a most powerful action as a relaxant and a normalizer of the female reproductive system. Active ingredients in the herb include resin, bitter glycosides, ranunculin—which changes to anemonin upon drying—salicylic acid, tannin and estrogenic principle.

"It may be used beneficially in cases of painful or delayed menstruation," says David Hoffmann in *The New Holistic Herbal*. "Ovarian cramps or cramping pain in the womb will be relieved by black cohosh. It has a normalizing action on the balance of female sex hormones and may safely be used to regain normal hormonal activity."

Black cohosh is very active in the treatment of rheumatic conditions of all kinds. It may be used in cases of rheumatic pain, in rheumatoid arthritis, osteoarthritis, in muscular and neurological pain, sciatica and neuralgia.

As a relaxing nervine, black cohosh may be used in many situations were such an agent is needed. It will be useful in labor to aid uterine activity while allaying nervousness. It will reduce spasm and thus aid in the treatment of pulmonary complaints such as whooping cough. It has also been found beneficial in cases of tinnitus.

CLINICAL STUDIES

In gynecology, black cohosh is currently being used to treat functional disorders of the female genitals and the concomitant autonomic symptoms which are linked to it as a result of a disturbed hormonal mechanism during the menarche and in menopause, according to *Notebene Medici* in 1980. Researchers reported an improvement in such symptoms as hot flashes, palpitations of the heart, restlessness, headaches, ringing in the ears, sleep disturbances and depressive mood swings. In fact, all cases of mild hormonal dysfunction, especially in older women, could be relieved with *cimicifuga* alone, and only in about 20 percent of the cases was it necessary to use additional hormone therapy.

On average, the treatment with black cohosh extract lasted from three to six months. Tolerance of the preparation was said to be excellent, and, even in long-term therapy, there were no specific side effects or unphysiological bleeding. The researchers, therefore, categorized black cohosh as an effective and low-risk alternative to the currently common and often criticized estrogen or estrogen-androgen therapy in the treatment of menstrual and menopausal complaints.

In a study reported in *Planta Medica* in 1991, Eva-Maria Dueker, et al., of the University of Göttingen in Germany, reiterated that cessation of ovarian function during menopause is characterized by reduced estrogen production and increased LH and FSH secretion. These endocrine changes result in hot flashes, depression, etc., which are usually treated with estrogen. However, although estrogen replacement is a suitable therapy, there is a need for alternative treatments, since women often refuse to take steroid hormone replacement or because such therapies are contraindicated.

Their study involved 110 women, who had not received steroid replacement therapy for at least six months and who complained of the typical symptoms facing menopausal women. The mean age of the volunteers was 52 plus or minus two years. Half of the women were given two tablets daily of Remifemin, each containing 2 mg of a dried extract of the rhizome of *Cimicifuga racemosa*, which yielded 4 mg extract per day. After two months of treatment, a blood sample was taken in the morning and LH and FSH were measured by commercially available LH and FSH radioimmunoassay kits.

Following the two-month study with Remifemin, the researchers stated that LH levels were significantly reduced in comparison with the women given a placebo. However, FSH levels in both treatment groups were similar.

The research team pointed out that hot flashes are the most common symptoms associated with menopause, and that they affect 75 percent of menopausal women. There is evidence, they said, that hot flashes, as measured objectively by increased skin temperature, coincide with the occurrence of LH episodes.

"We have evidence that a pharmaceutical preparation of *Cimicifuga racemosa* (known as Remifemin) is able to suppress LH secretion in menopausal women," the researchers said. "Since pulsatile LH secretion and the occurrence of hot flashes are closely related, measurement of LH levels is a suitable parameter to study the potency of plant extracts in regard to the reduction of hot flashes. To the best of our knowledge, this is the first report about a plant extract affecting LH secretion in both humans and [rats]."

In a report in *Medwelt* in 1985, G. Warnecke, M.D. said that the endocrine changes during menopause, especially estrogen deficiency, lead to a series of somatic, psychological and neurovegetative symptoms, which are compounded by psychosocial and cultural factors in addition to the aging process. The neurovegetative (involuntary hormone system) dysfunctional symptoms are most apparent in the early menopause, and they last for more than a year in 80 percent of the women and over five years in 33 percent of the women. This is accompanied by atrophic-inflammatory mucosal processes, so that the attending physician is faced with the task of conducting his/her therapy over a number of years and adjusting it to the severity of the symptoms and the main symptom prevailing at any time, Warnecke said.

"For some time," he continued, "it has been possible to determine a transformation of the recognized hormonal therapy of menopausal symptoms among the patients concerned. Many of these women spontaneously express the wish not to be treated with chemicals or even hormones under any circumstances. The orientation towards a more biological therapy of menopausal symptoms, perhaps set off by the media or by reports that certain drugs were being withdrawn from the market, is becoming increasingly noticeable in medical practice."

Among the physiological substances available for the treatment of menopausal symptoms, a standardized extract of Cimicifuga has particular proven its worth, he said. He referred to an animal experiment on ovariectomied rats to determine the endocrine efficacy of the constituents of Remifemin, and it was shown that the extract not only reduces the secretion of the pituitary hormone LH, but also competes with estradiol for estrogen receptors.

Warnecke's study involved 60 women, ranging in age from 40 to 60 years old, who were being treated in a gynecology practice. The patients were randomly assigned to three groups, and they were admitted to the study only if they had no or only irregular bleeding and complained of menopausal symptoms that did not require high-dose hormone treatment or special therapy with psychotropic drugs from the outset.

During the 12-week study, 20 women were given 50 drops of Remifemin (equivalent to two tablets); 20 were treated with 0.6 mg of conjugated estrogens and the remaining 20 received 2 mg/day of diazepam. The investigations were conducted at the beginning of the study and after two, four and 12 weeks of treatment.

Eighty percent of the women had already entered menopause, and compliance was good in almost all cases, with only isolated cases of irregular intake, Warnecke reported. Five of the volunteers dropped out of the study, two on hormone treatment after eight and 10 weeks; two on the psychotropic drug after eight and 11 weeks, and one on Remifemin after 10 weeks. An improvement in the menopausal symptoms was basically achieved in all three therapies.

Warnecke reported that a long-term and consistent therapy of menopausal symptoms with Remifemin yields rates of success at least equivalent to low-dose conjugated estrogen and better ones than therapy with psychotropic drugs. The latter only treats the autonomic and psychological alterations and, as expected, no changes in the somatic parameters could be determined on psychotropic drugs.

"Since the majority of women with menopausal symptoms are usually affected by the spectrum of mild to moderate dysfunctional symptoms, a therapeutic approach with Remifemin is basically justified," Warnecke said, "especially when one takes into account the risks of long-term therapy with hormones and psychotropic drugs. The overall results obtained with Remifemin in this study are outstanding."

As a basic rule, he added, one should attempt to achieve the optimum effect with the lowest-risk therapy. The advantages of this phytotherapeutic agent are its outstanding spectrum of action in the climacteric syndrome, the absence of toxic side effects and thus the possibility of long-term therapy. In mild and moderate menopausal dysfunctional symptoms, preference should, therefore, be given to the phytotherapeutic agent Remifemin as the substance of first choice. The use of Remifemin is particularly indicated in all cases in which treatment with hormones or psychotropic drugs is contraindicated, as well as in women who state a preference for a biological therapy from the outset, he said.

Warnecke concluded by saying that in no way should any

warranted therapy with animal sex hormones be made superfluous, but an often satisfactory therapeutic response can undoubtedly be achieved by the systematic use of physiological, hormonelike substances. The mechanism of action of individual physiological drug extracts on the endocrine system has already been thoroughly researched, but often remains practically unknown. Research into active substances from medicinal plants is both interesting and promising, even in this era of enormous development of chemical substances.

Fifty women, ranging in age from 45 to 60, all having menopausal complaints, were treated with Remifemin by G. Vorberg, M.D., a physician in Munich, Germany, in an open, unpublished study. Thirty-nine patients showed contraindications to hormone therapy: thrombosis, phlebitis, varicosis, diabetes, endometriosis, etc. Eleven of the patients refused hormone replacement therapy.

Vorberg noted that the improvement of the somatic findings, the neurovegetative and psychic symptoms and signs were significant or even highly significant. Each volunteer received 40 drops/day (equivalent to two tablets) of Remifemin. Four of the patients reported slight gastrointestinal problems at the beginning of the study, but otherwise there were no prominent side effects while using Remifemin, Vorberg said.

After four weeks of therapy with Remifemin, Vorberg reported a significant decrease in hot flashes, sweating, nervousness, irritability and headache. By the end of the twelfth week, most of the symptoms, except lack of concentration and arthritic pains, had eased.

The *Cimicifuga racemosa* (Remifemin) lessened the extent of hot flashes, sweating and insomnia in 36 women observed by W. Daiber, M.D., a German physician, he reported in *Arztliche Praxis* in 1983. The volunteers received 40 drops (equivalent to two tablets) twice a day of Remifemin for 12 weeks.

"A hormone-free alternative treatment is needed for women in whom this therapy is contraindicated or for women who refuse to be treated with hormones," Daiber said. "With Remifemin there is available a phytogenic preparation which possesses an excellent compatibility and a high effectiveness. The fact that the effect does not take place as rapidly as in the use of hormone therapy is compensated for by its excellent compatibility and the possibility of long-term administration. A habit-forming or dependence, as often found with psychotropic drugs, does not materialize with Remifemin."

He added that physicians, in treating menopausal women, should be aware of the possibility of endometrial cancer when estrogen replacement therapy is prescribed, therefore, an initial hormone-free treatment is of great use to many women and it does not harm anyone.

Writing in *Der Landarzt* in 1958, Ernst Wolrad Schotten, M.D. reported that he had been prescribing Remifemin for almost a year. He gave his patients 20 drops (equivalent to 1 tablet) of the extract three times a day and noted that it does not kick in immediately, but does so after a relatively short time. Giving this therapy for three to four weeks was so successful that he was able to reduce the dose to 10 drops three times a day. He found it remarkable that he was able to stop administration of the originally required sedatives, due to the calming effect, particularly on the psyche. A normalization of fluctuating blood pressure was also observed.

"Depression clearly subsided and complete freedom from symptoms often occurred," he observed. "Above all, the patients repeatedly stressed the mildly euphoric effect of the product. By tailoring the dosage of each individual patient, most of them were able to continue working. If present, even joint troubles receded."

He recorded a very favorable effect on premenstrual phenomena accompanied by subjective, general circulatory symptoms, without menstruation being artificially induced. In addition to the indications mentioned, he noted an exceptionally good toleration and sedative effect in women with pregnancy complaints that led to their inability to work. Even if vomiting could not be eliminated entirely, the calming effect was so strong that all other sedatives could be discontinued. The results of the 22 patients that he observed over six months displayed a marked improvement, and the preparation had at least a psychologically calming effect in the rest of the cases.

"I would like to stress that the principle *nil nocere* ['do no harm'] continues to apply in this therapy, while symptoms that occur in the two important stages of a woman's life—before menarche and the beginning of menopause—can be very favorably influenced without intervening heavy-handedly in the hormonal metabolism and pituitary processes," Schotten said. "The product should definitely be administered at a gradually increasing dose and over a longer period for the treatment of hormonal transitional symptoms. The effect sets in slowly but is all the more sustained. Patients who do not respond—and this naturally cannot be ruled out—should be placed in the hands of a specialist."

In an essay in 1960, A. Bruecker, M.D., said that, on the basis of four years of experience with 517 female patients, he concluded that Cimicifuga extract has a hormonelike and slightly euphoric effect. This beneficial effect is particularly evident in autonomic-psychic change-of-life phenomena in the various age groups. There is no risk of adverse side effects, particularly no unphysiological bleeding, he said.

"It is generally recommended that greater attention be paid to phytotherapy for controlling mild and moderate cases in menopausal women in order to reduce the use of potent substances, especially hormones."

Bruecker reviewed a number of case histories that had been published in 1960. Dosage of Remifemin was usually 20 to 30 drops or one tablet three times a day over a rather long period. Since the effect of the treatment is often delayed, short-term use of the product is pointless. The drops should be retained as long as possible in the mouth and the tablets sucked on.

"Remifemin alone was able to improve dysfunctional symptoms and autonomic disorders in 79 percent of the women who still had ovarian activity. In cases of total ovariectomy, it was possible to reduce the use of hormones considerably by the supplementary administration of Remifemin. The interval between long-acting hormone injections could thus be increased from three to eight weeks."

Bruecker added that there have been individual cases in which a marked improvement in depression was observed following Remifemin therapy. The product also appeared to have a stronger effect on the psyche than did sex hormones.

He referred to one group of patients with predominantly autonomic symptoms. Some of the women were sexually mature, but usually the patients were going through menopause. There were good results with Remifemin, including the control of circulatory symptoms. In two patients who had had their ovaries removed, mild menstrual bleeding was observed. But premenstrual symptoms such as listlessness, anxiety, hot flashes and general complaints during pregnancy also benefited from the use of Remifemin, and no detrimental effect on the pregnancy was observed.

Another German researcher, A. Petho, M.D., in an unpublished paper, discussed his experience in which menopausal women who were receiving hormone injections were switched to Remifemin. In 50 percent of the patients pretreated by hormones, they no longer needed the injections after receiving the black cohosh preparation.

The study involved 50 volunteers who had been receiving the hormone injections for various menopausal complaints. After being prescribed Remifemin for six months, 28 patients no longer needed the injections; 21 patients required one injection; one patient needed two injections. The gynecologist reported that Remifemin produced very good results in 21 patients, good results in 20 patients and a minor effect in nine patients. There were no side effects with the Remifemin therapy.

Petho noted that substances in *Cimicifuga racemosa* bind to estrogen receptors, reducing the secretion of the luteinizing hormone (LH) without influencing the pituitary release of follicle-stimulating hormone (FSH) or prolactin. The extract works slowly over a period of weeks, therefore, the treatment can be prolonged at the physician's discretion.

The researcher determined that the active principles in the black cohosh preparation included triterpene glycosides (cimicifugoside, cimigenol, 27-deoxyactein, etc.) and isoflavones (e.g., formononetin). It is believed that the triterpene derivatives act directly on the hypothalamic-pituitary system. Effects of cimicifuga extract on the vagus and vasomotor centers have also been reported.

"So far, our experiences prove the effectiveness of the cimicifuga treatment and the graduated withdrawal of a hormone therapy," Petho continued. "Our study shows that the therapeutic response was maintained in most cases, even when there was a change-over from estrogen-androgen injections to Remifemin. Unwanted side effects could not be observed at any time. It should be kept in mind that the full efficacy of the cimicifuga extract is not evident for several weeks, so the therapy should last for at least six months. If the indications of pre- and postmenopausal syndrome are carefully defined, it is our impression that the administration of Remifemin can be regarded as a valuable addition to the therapeutic arsenal."

In a double-blind study, not yet published, Wolfgang Stoll, M.D. assigned volunteers at random to three groups: 1) 30 patients were given two tablets, containing 2 mg of 27-deoxyactein standardized from cimicifuga dry extract, twice daily; 2) 30 patients received one tablet containing 0.625 mg conjugated estrogenic substances plus three placebo tablets daily for 21 days. After that they were given placebo tablets daily for seven days; 3) 20 patients were given two placebo tablets twice daily.

Three parameters were kept in mind during the study: 1) The menopausal index according to Kupperman, which measured mainly neurovegetative symptoms; 2) the Hamilton anxiety scale for psychological complaints; and 3) the proliferation status of vaginal epithelium as an objective parameter. The first two criteria were investigated every four weeks; the third was evaluated at the beginning of the study and at the end after 12 weeks.

"After three months of therapy with the phytotherapeuticon, all three parameters had significantly improved," Stoll said. "The estrogen dose proved to be too low, and it yielded no effect compared to placebo. However, the usefulness of Remifemin as an alternative to estrogen could be substantiated."

He added that the gynecologist has to consider the risk-benefit of hormone replacement therapy for menopausal complaints, and that an effective alternative is available in the Remifemin herbal remedy.

Another German researcher, Helga Stolze, M.D., said that the hormone-free Remifemin can be seen as an alternative to hormones and psychoactive drugs. This standardized extract of the black cohosh root is able to improve or, at least, to remove partially menopausal complaints because a regulation of the ovarian function, as well as of the autonomic nervous system, is obtained without using hormones. Because of available experimental test results, the preparation's main site of action is a control system of the ovaries, probably the anterior pituitary gland, she said.

"The results of treatment with Remifemin documented on 1,738 patients in clinical and general practice prove that this preparation improves the symptoms and signs of the menopausal complaints, including neurovegetative disturbances, i.e., a gradual regulation of the hormonal balance is obtained. In many cases, even slight postoperative deficiency symptoms could be removed using Remifemin, and in only 20 percent of the cases was additional hormone therapy necessary. However, the dose could be reduced due to the Remifemin treatment."

Stolze added that Remifemin can be considered an alternative in the treatment of menopausal complaints in those cases where a treatment with estrogens or psychotropic drugs is not indicated because of the risks and side effects associated with hormone therapy, or, in general, a specific medication is not necessary. Besides the documented efficacy—improvements in 80 percent of the patients—the advantage of Remifemin in therapeutic practice is that the preparation, unlike estrogens and psychoactive drugs, can be applied without hesitation within the scope of a long-term therapy because of its excellent tolerance.

OTHER USES FOR REMIFEMIN

Although Remifemin is perhaps best known for alleviating the symptoms of menopause (hot flashes, etc.), it has and is being used for a variety of gynecological complaints.

Writing in *Ringelh. Biol. Umsch.* in 1964, Eugen Schildge, M.D. said that he had been using Remifemin in his practice for many years to treat girls and women. The product was useful not only in menopausal depressive states, but also for premenstrual syndrome (PMS) symptoms.

"Besides mood brightening in the sense of mild euphoria, Remifemin relaxes and calms the patient," he said. "It was particularly this euphoric and relaxant effect that, in my opinion, has led to Remifemin becoming a good agent used in neurological practice to treat such psychological symptoms."

He referred to the work of Goerlich, who has described his experience with Remifemin in the diversity of manifestations seen in his gynecological practice. In his opinion, the autonomic-endocrine syndrome in the woman has a rigidly outlined clinical picture which is characterized by lack of vasostability, constipation and ovarian insufficiency. He discussed 88 cases in which the patients complained of cold feet and hands, headache, dizziness, cramping, constipation and fluctuations in the monthly period. He gave the women one-half of one Remifemin tablet twice a day and found that, over time, he was able to observe that the autonomic symptoms either subsided or disappeared. The gradual improvement in general well-being was remarkable. Sleep improved and the disturbances of vasostability were also eliminated.

For his PMS patients, Schildge prescribes 20 drops (equivalent to 1 tablet) of Remifemin three times a day for three to six months and, depending on the effect, he converts to "interval therapy" from the 15th day after the period starts until menstruation has begun again. However, in the case of menopausal depressive states, chronic medication of 30 drops (equivalent to 1-2 tablets) three times a day without interruption is indicated. The patients invariably improve with this therapy, he said.

He described the case of a 17-year-old clerk who regularly experienced PMS nine days before the start of menses, resulting in fatigue, low spirits, insomnia, tingling in the hands, a stale taste while eating, etc. She improved gradually following two months on Remifemin. After four months, it was possible to convert to an interval treatment, and she was able to work during the premenstrual phase.

"In a total of 135 cases of premenstrual and menopausal mood swings and depressive states, Remifemin performed very well. The improvement in general well-being resulting from the mild euphoric and relaxant-sedative effect was remarkable. An average dose of 20 drops (equivalent to 1 tablet) of Remifemin t.i.d. [three times a day] over a period of three to six months was prescribed which, under certain circumstances for chronic therapy, could be lowered to 10 drops t.i.d. The product was always well tolerated."

K. Stiehler, M.D., reporting in *Arztliche Praxis* in 1959, said that, based on a number of studies, it is often possible to eliminate symptoms associated with menopause and dysfunction after hysterectomy without ovariectomy with Remifemin. On the other hand, in the first and second year of menopause and after hysterectomy and ovariectomy, it is useful to combine Remifemin with small doses of follicular hormones by prescribing a dose of the common hormone products in the mornings and 20 drops (equivalent to 1 tablet) of Remifemin at noontime and in the evenings, and then gradually converting to Remifemin medication exclusively.

In an article in *Arztliche Praxis* in 1962, N. Goerlich, M.D. reviewed his protocol in the treatment of ovarian disorders. In 41 of 49 patients with PMS, he was able to eradicate such symptoms as mood swings, circulatory disorders and headaches which occurred about one week before menstruation with Remifemin. If 20 drops, or one tablet, of Remifemin were given three times daily 12 to 14 days before menstruation, the typical symptoms did not surface.

Dysmenorrhea is a condition in which women experience abdominal and lower back pain during menstruation and after it ends. Instead of analgesics and sedatives, he prescribes 10 drops or one-half tablet of Remifemin three times daily between the 10th and 20th day of the menstrual cycle. In 16 of 24 cases, he found that the women confronted their menstrual cramps more calmly and objectively, complained less, and continued working without mishap. They did have some pain—Remifemin is not an analgesic—but the symptoms were generally not as strident as before therapy.

"Remifemin alone is not sufficient in dysmenorrhea, but I did see very good results in so-called ovulation or intermediate pain. Those unpleasant, tearing pains when the follicle bursts no longer occur if one Remifemin tablet is taken four times daily between the 10th and 14th day over several periods. Apparently, Remifemin effectively slows the sudden drop in estrogen production occurring around this time."